How to Smoke Pot:

The Beginners Guide for Legalized Marijuana

By David Reagan

To get free alerts on up to date
changes to law, new products,
and other important information
join the email list at:

www.WeedBookClub.com

David@WeedBookClub.com

The Forward

In the last several years, few topics have been as hotly debated in the United States as marijuana. Reform movements have taken hold across the country, spawning a booming legal industry flush with entrepreneurs cashing in on everything from pot cookies to marijuana-infused lube. Even in some states holding tight to restrictive laws, discussions about relaxing criminal penalties for low-level marijuana offenses are afoot.

It's the product of decades of pro-marijuana politicking. Yes, hired lobbyists troll the hallways of Congress and state legislatures. Recreational or medical marijuana is now legal in 23 states and Washington, DC. And every November voters somewhere in the country cast a new round of ballots weighing in on the issue.

Despite a steady groundswell of support at the state level, marijuana remains illegal at the federal level, though the Obama administration has signaled a willingness to tolerate what states are doing so long as local officials strictly enforce regulations.

So, what does all this mean? In the simplest form: you can now enjoy marijuana legally in some parts of the country. But there's still a lot to know before your first smoke or your first visit to a pot shop.

I decided to explore this topic a bit more on a recent trip, immersing myself in several eye-opening visits to dispensaries across Denver. What I found was quite amazing.

Admittedly, I would have considered myself a novice in this world before the Denver trip. That has changed, and I'd like to share some of what I've learned along the way to help you as a newbie navigating marijuana culture for the first time.

Full disclosure: My interest in the topic stems from a trip to Amsterdam a few years ago, where I first experimented with marijuana. It was great. But I couldn't quite achieve the same results back home. I've come to learn it's all about the details: the strain, the quality of the grow operation and, maybe most importantly, personal preferences when it comes to the overall experience.

From my perspective, the dispensary process was easy, clean, and friendly. And it was fairly straightforward. Once inside a pot shop, it can best be described as similar to an Apple-store experience: chic retail ambiance, lush green product stored in large containers on sleek display tables and in some cases there are even tablets to provide information on specific strains.

I put this book together to pass along the basics for your own trip to a dispensary, to understand the risks, the ways to enjoy pot, where it's legal, how to cook it, some of the varieties available and what to look for to make your experience more enjoyable.

Welcome to Marijuana 101 – why wasn't this offered in college?

Marijuana 101[1]

Marijuana. Hemp. Pot. Grass. Hashish. are some of the many names that you will hear cannabis referred to. Hemp comes from the cannabis plant but is strictly used in an industrial manner for clothes, rope, paper and building materials. That's to say — you don't smoke the stuff.

Hashish, or hash, is an extremely potent cannabis product usually mixed with marijuana or tobacco. It's made from dried resin glands, called trichomes that come from the leaves and flowers of the plant, and is compressed into a finished product that usually looks like brown chunks. It's most commonly found in the Middle East and North Africa. Some dispensaries in Colorado carry hash in its original form but not all. Hash oils and other extracts, however, are generally available at most dispensaries.

Other parts cannabis of the plant are used to create oils and other forms of the drug. Sometimes these oils are used to make edibles, like hash brownies, and other treats that can be baked. The ingredient that gets you high in the is a compound called tetrahydrocannabinol or THC. Most dispensaries will measure and display the estimated THC level of a specific strain so you can gauge potency — the higher the THC count the stronger the strain.

Types of Weed and Their Effects[1]

There are two main things to consider when it comes to a marijuana high.

1. The effects will depend on the strain you are smoking (more on that below).

2. How the marijuana is grown and where it is cultivated will also play major roles in determining potency, flavor and price.

Another thing to consider: Eating marijuana has a long-lasting effect, ranging anywhere from four to 10 hours and produces more of a body high, where as smoking marijuana can keep you buzzed for about three hours. But it varies based on individual tolerance and what you're smoking.

There are two main subspecies of cannabis: indica and sativa. Legal marijuana sold in stores will be classified as one or the other. Growers have also crossbred strains with both subspecies to create a large number of hybrids. One strain is preferable for an uplifting high, while the other is more prone to what stoners call "couch lock."

Indica: Indica varieties are known to come from southern Asia and near India (think Afghanistan, Pakistan, India, Tibet and Nepal). Indicas plants are dense and stocky, with heavy, dense, fragrant buds. The effect of an Indica is generally centered more on the body and classified as a 'heavy stone'. It is common to heighten physical sensations such as touch, taste and sound. It has a relaxing effect - mentally and physically - and is generally recommended if someone is having problems sleeping.

Sativa: Sativas generally from the warmer regions, near the equator - Thailand, Cambodia, Jamaica, and Mexico. Sativas are known for their 'uplifting high' that can be characterized as cerebral, creative, energetic, giggly and sometimes   even psychedelic. It is less overpowering than the high produced by an Indica.

Within these two subspecies of cannabis, growers have spawned no shortage of individual marijuana strains, each with its own smell, flavor and potency. Some of the more popular strains include Ak47, White Rhino, NYC Diesel, Girl Scout Cookies, White Widow, Blueberry and Northern Lights. There are literally hundreds of other strains, and if you buy weed with a specific name you can do a search at www.mjguide.com or at Leafly.com.

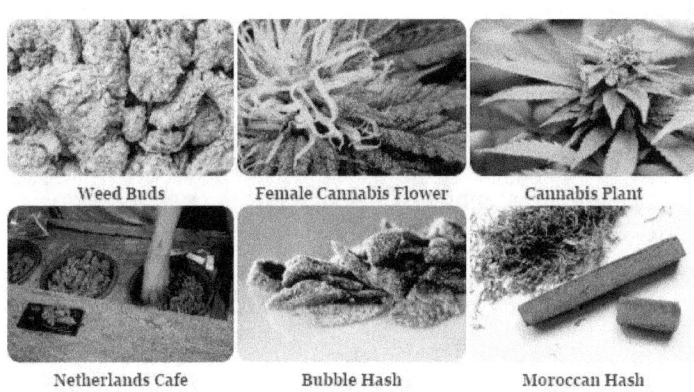

| Weed Buds | Female Cannabis Flower | Cannabis Plant |
| Netherlands Cafe | Bubble Hash | Moroccan Hash |

Picture from: Website Title: Buzzle Article Title: Different Types of Weed and Their Effects

Qualities2

Slang tends to vary by location. I will go over the fairly universal word below to help to describe the quality of weed. A complete guide of marijuana terminology is also available at the back of this book.

Schwag: This is basically crap weed. It is brown, seedy, and usually dry. Schwag is very cheap, generally moved into the United States from Mexico, in some cases in a gas tank. You'll never see this type of stuff in a legal pot shop.

Mids: This is middle of the road weed. This weed will be much prettier and will smell and taste better than schwag, depending on where it is purchased. There will also be fewer seeds. This stuff is not sold in dispensaries either.

Dank: Main physical attributes: Plenty of crystals, red, gold or pretty yellow hairs, a beautiful green color, dense nugs, pungent aroma and no seeds. This is the stuff you're looking to buy at a dispensary. It is often sold in medicine bottles for easy storing.

Quantities

Weed quantities are fairly standard. It is sold in ounces or grams usually. This is how you will experience it in a legal dispensary.

1/8 (of an ounce) "eight": 3.5 grams
1/4 (of an ounce) "quarter/q": 7 grams
1/2 (of an ounce) "half": 14 grams
1 ounce: "O.Z." 28 grams
quarter-pound: "Q.P" 4 ounces

Prices will vary depending on what state you are in and the laws outlining marijuana sale and use. In Colorado, where pot is legal, one ounce of super-potent marijuana can sell for as low as $125. But in most states where the drug is still prohibited, the cost of one-eight of an ounce tends to average $50 to $60 and a full ounce can go for about $400.

Selecting Joint Rolling Papers
There are plenty of brands of rolling papers. Some of the most popular are JOBs or Zig-Zags. You should be able to find them in most gas stations. In Europe, a brand called Rizla is popular.

Rice-based Papers: These work very nice. Rice-based papers are super thin and have almost no taste, giving you maximum ability to extract actual flavor from your marijuana smoke. I recommend a brand called Elements. One thing to note: since rice papers are so thin, they can be more difficult to roll with.

Ways To Smoke

Joint – A mix of weed and hash rolled up in a paper.

Spliff – A joint rolled with tobacco and weed

Roach – The tail end of a joint.

Blunt - Weed (and/or hash) rolled in cigar paper. There are pre-packaged blunt rolling papers, but a lot of people buy cheap commercial cigars, like a Phillie Blunt or a Swisher Sweets, slice it open and remove the tobacco. The emptied cigar wrapper is then rolled with weed.

Dry Pipes – Smoking from a pipe is usually called "hitting a bowl" because you pack the weed in the end if the pipe in a bowl shaped space. These pipes do not use water. Pipes can be made of all sorts of materials, including soda cans or an apple if you're desperate or crafty, but the safest and preferred material is glass. A high quality glass piece, one built to withstand, is an expensive but worthwhile investment.

There are several different types of dry pipes:
1. **Chillum** – Often called one hitters -These are tiny pipes with very little bowls only good for one or two hits. They have straight shafts. The weed goes at the top, and you inhale smoke from the bottom. They are compact, easy to hide and also very convenient for sneaking a toke in public.

2. **Spoon** - Spoons are relatively inexpensive and good value for the price. You can always buy a very expensive exotic one. Spoons range in size — there are huge ones but generally they are fairly smallest pipe you will find, though chillums are larger

3. **Sherlock** - Named for Sherlock Holmes, these pipes are characterized by a curved neck.

Color-changing glass: One of the most popular is the glass pipe that can change color with use, providing different hues over time depending on how the glass is blown.

Water Pipes – These are used to filter the smoke through the water, which cools the temperature of the smoke which allows for a cleaners and smooth hit. Sometimes people will use other liquids other than water.

Wet pipes:

1. **Bubbler** - Basically a type of water pipe, but you will hear this term. These are pipes with a chamber attached under the bowl that can be filled with water. Chamber sizes range, but the bigger the chamber the more water you can put in.

2. **Bong** - Officially referred to as a water pipe if you're in a head shop, this is the king of smoking accessories. Bongs work just like bubblers but they have bigger chambers for water. Bongs tend to stand upright and can be large – some measuring up to 6 feet in extreme cases.

Health Effects of Smoking Weed[3]

According to the National Institute on Drug Abuse, marijuana smoke contains cancer causing substances. Some research shows that marijuana smoke has up to 70% more cancer causing ingredients than tobacco smoke.

According to some studies, smoking marijuana produces a nearly three-fold increase of inhaled tar compared to tobacco. This is probably because of the lack of filter. Other research suggests that marijuana smokers, compared to cigarette smokers, often inhale more deeply and hold their breath longer, to get more effect from the THC. Finally, according to a 2012 study in the Journal of the American Medical Association it appears light users of marijuana does cause loss of lung function,

Long-term, heavy use of marijuana can lead to impaired thinking skills and memory problems.
- There is some level of scientific debate over the link between marijuana and schizophrenia
- Potential for anxiety, depression or lethargy.
- Marijuana is addictive and once a person stops using, the withdrawal symptoms, along with intensity, will vary from person to person. Withdrawal symptoms can last anywhere from days to weeks and include restlessness, crankiness, anxiety, stomach pain, loss of appetite, aggression and sleeping problems.

Health Benefits of Marijuana:

Marijuana is at the center of a quickly evolving medical field. Used in most cases to help ease chronic pain or to stimulate appetite in terminally ill patients, doctors are exploring w   ith marijuana to treat patients suffering from conditions like asthma, Parkinson's disease, alcohol abuse, anorexia, depression, arthritis, epilepsy, sleep apnea, and glaucoma.

Marijuana can also provide relief for patients suffering from health conditions like breast and brain cancer, multiple sclerosis and AIDS.

When you get high, what are some of the basic physical reactions you can expect?

Some Natural Reactions:
- Dry mouth
- Blood pressure hike
- Increased appetite
- Rapid breathing
- Reddened eyes
- Slow reflexes
- Lethargy

Good Reactions:
- Heightened sense of smell, touch, and hearing
- Relaxed state of being
- Giggly feeling
- Increased libido
- Increased empathy
- Physical pain relief
- Reduced anxiety

Bad Reactions:
- Bad withdrawal symptoms for heavy users
- Increased heart rate
- Anxiety
- Addiction
- Exposure to contaminants used to grow marijuana. An array of chemicals, including pesticides, is used to grow marijuana. And those chemicals are not listed on the container of weed at your local dispensary, so that means you have no real idea what kind of chemicals you're smoking unless you've developed a relationship with a grower.

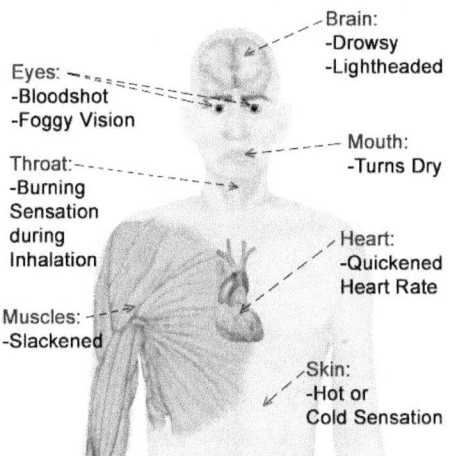

Brain:
-Drowsy
-Lightheaded

Eyes:
-Bloodshot
-Foggy Vision

Mouth:
-Turns Dry

Throat:
-Burning
Sensation
during
Inhalation

Heart:
-Quickened
Heart Rate

Muscles:
-Slackened

Skin:
-Hot or
Cold Sensation

Picture from: Website Title: Buzzle Article Title: Different Types of Weed and Their Effects

Vaporizer[4]

Touted as the healthiest way to inhale marijuana, vaporizing is the process of heating marijuana to about 380°F to 410° F, just below the point of combustion. The result is pure THC vapor, not smoke, that is free of damaging carcinogens and the onslaught of other nasty materials that stem from combustion, i.e. igniting marijuana with a flame and generating smoke to inhale.

Vaporizers used to be big, clumsy looking contraptions, most notably characterized by a plastic bag that fit over the top. In recent years, vaporizers have evolved into slick, compact mobile gadgets, paving a path for an entire market revolving around high-end vape devices. One of the most popular is called the Ploom Pax, which retails for about $250 online.

By and large, mobile vaporizers are increasingly becoming one of the most prominent go-to devices for marijuana use.

Cannabis Concentrates

The future of cannabis consumption is steadily steering toward potent concentrated forms of the drug. Concentrates refer to the final product produced by using a solvent — like butane, ethanol or CO_2 — to extract resin glands from the plant matter.

Hash is the oldest form of a concentrate, but nowadays concentrates encompass everything from wax or dabs to tinctures placed under your tongue to hash and butane oil smoked via vape pen.

These concentrates can be up to 80% HC, compared to some of the most marijuana flower strains that clock in at around 20 percent to 25 percent. So keep in mind these are extremely potent.

Edibles[5]

Marijuana-infused edibles are another popular way to enjoy the drug. Cooking with marijuana has moved well beyond just pot brownies, and dispensaries now are doing a booming trade in cookbooks, savory pot foods and frozen takeout dishes that incorporate the drug.

Legalization of marijuana has also led to somewhat of a revolution in terms of making pot-infused food safer.

There's actual lab testing of edibles happening to help determine dosages and potency for commercial use. And most dispensaries nowadays have their edibles, be it gummy worms or candy bars, labeled with the THC content listed in milligrams.

Take it easy when dealing with edibles. It's not hard to over do it. But there are consequences. Eating an overdose of THC is something even a seasoned smoker tries to avoid.

Everyone's metabolism is different but about 10 milligrams to 25 milligrams of THC will make your muscles relax and will induce a general wave of bliss throughout your entire body. Giggling can be common, and you will feel very relaxed. The high can last from four to six hours, or longer with higher doses.

Also important to note: THC is insoluble in water but soluble in fats, oil and alcohol. That means you will have to extract the THC from the marijuana into a butter — "cannabutter"— or an oil — "cannaoil"— and use that for cooking.

Since THC is soluble in alcohol, another effective way of adding it into dishes is through cooking brandy or rum infused with cannabinoids.

The culinary potential is almost limitless so long as you take heed to a couple of simple rules. One of the most important is making sure to cook your edibles at a temperature that never exceeds 300 degrees Fahrenheit.

General tips for dealing with edibles:

1. Do not eat on empty stomach: You should treat edibles like you would a painkiller — like Percocet or Vicodin. Maybe start with a little bit, and have it with some food. You want to avoid having it on an empty stomach

2. Measuring by milligrams: 10 milligrams tend to be the standard dose of THC. For instance if there is a 100-milligram chocolate bar splits into 10 pieces, each one is roughly 10 milligrams apiece. Dose accordingly. It's important.

3. Different brands, different consistency: Just like medicine people react differently. Some people have a different reaction or e xperience with infused gummies or infused chocolates. Experiment with different brands. Find what you like. Again, ask your bud tender and friends.

4. The waiting game: This is important for first time users. For people who don't have high tolerances, 10-20 milligrams is a good place to start, especially with edibles, because you don't want to ingest too much. So start slow, and wait 45 minutes after you take it to see how you feel. You can always take more — but you can't go back and take less. Some edibles take longer than 45 minutes to kick in.

What to do if I eat too much?
Eating too much marijuana-infused food can be quite intense for some people. You may feel confused, sick, and even unable to move or talk. Remember your coordination may be heavily affected as well. If you eat too much and you feel the effects are too strong, you can try:

1. Eat citrus acid fruits such as lemons, oranges or grapefruits, or their juice.
2. Eating pistachios or pine nuts will help.
3. Use pine essential oil topically or inhalation.
4. Use a product rich in CBD (cannabidiol).

Intro to cooking[6]

Cooking with Marijuana:

If you want to cook with weed you will need to make certain quantity of "Cannabutter" or "Bud Butter", which is then used as a replacement for standard butter. To prepare weed for cooking it has to be heated in some way to extract the THC. Eating weed won't work without preparation, because the human digestive system is unable to process THC directly. The way to extract the THC is to use fat (oil, butter, milk) because THC is fat soluble and not water soluble. So keep in mind it is impossible to get high from pot tea, for example, without adding some milk or oil.

How much weed do I use?

One difficulty of cooking with marijuana is understanding the strength, which is determined by quality and amount of the weed you use for the butter or oil. The basic rule of thumb is four sticks of butters to every once of

Ingredients

1/4 ounce cannabis buds, *finely ground*   1/2 cup (one stick) *salted butter*

To make cannamargarine, simply substitute margarine for butter.

marijuana (can be a mix of marijuana and trim, too). This will make a pretty potent butter, so if you want something lighter just tweak the recipe accordingly.

Equipment

1 x Grinder

1 x Medium Saucepan

1 x Wooden Ladle

1 x Spoon

1 x Metal Strainer

1 x Container (with a tight fitting lid)

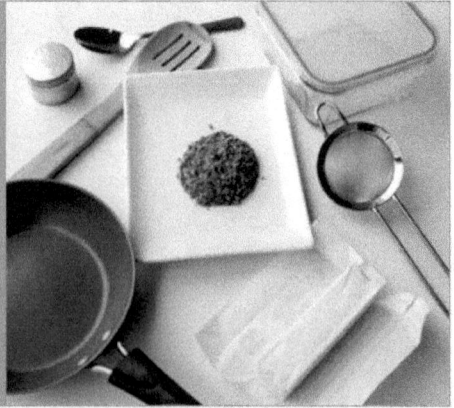

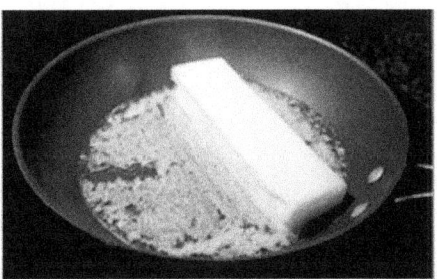

1 Melt the butter on low heat in a medium saucepan.

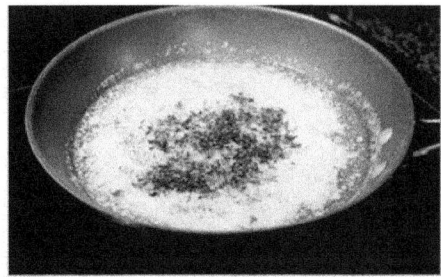

2 Add the ground buds to the melted butter a little bit at a time, stirring in between.

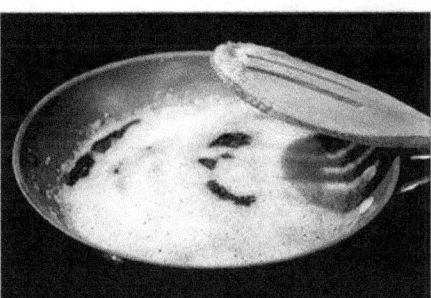

3 Simmer on a low heat for <u>45mins</u>, stirring frequently.

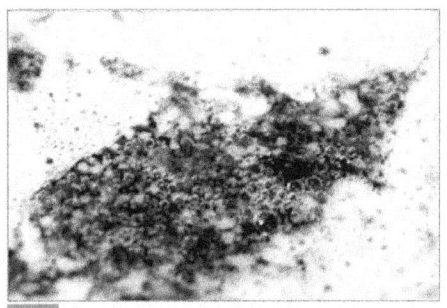

Tip You should see small bubbles slowly forming on the surface.

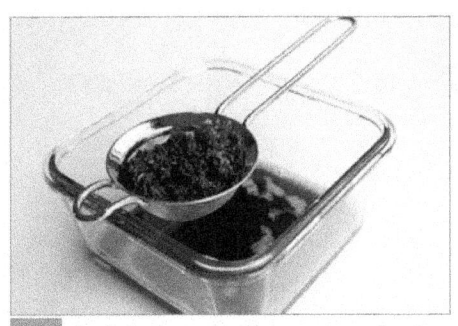

4 Strain the butter into the container using the metal strainer to filter out the ground buds.

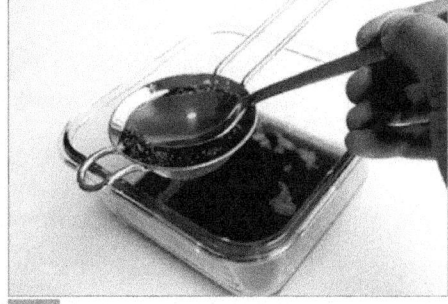

5 Press the spoon against the ground bud in the metal strainer to release all the cannabutter.

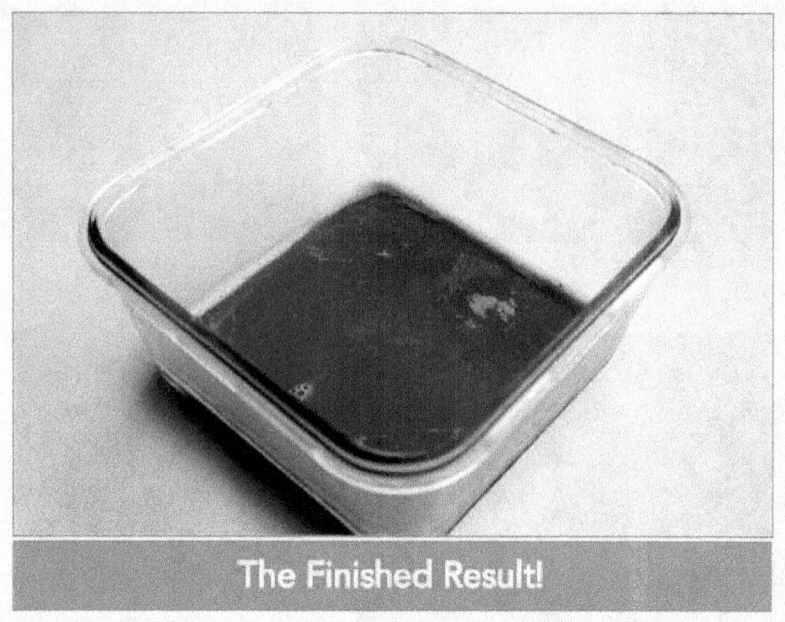

The Finished Result!

You can use the cannabutter immediately or
store it in the refrigerator for later.

Photos from: Website Title: How to Cook with Weed Article
Title: Cooking with weed

This recipe can easily scale up for larger batches. For
larger quantities we recommend that you simmer the butter
for 60 minutes, though some go even longer, to get the
maximum results.

*Note: For medical patients, we recommend using 2
ounces of cannabis for each pound of butter, effectively
doubling the strength of the cannabutter.*

Brownie Recipe[7]

Ingredients
- 1 cup all-purpose flour
- ¼ cup unsweetened cocoa powder
- ½ teaspoon baking powder
- ¼ teaspoon salt
- 3 tablespoons THC oil
- 5 ounces semisweet chocolate, chopped
- 1 ½ tablespoons light corn syrup
- 1 cup firmly packed light brown sugar
- 1 tablespoon applesauce
- 3 egg whites
- 2 teaspoons vanilla

Directions
Preheat oven to 275° Fahrenheit.(CAUTION NOT TO COOK AT TOO HIGH A TEMP)
1. In a small bowl, mix together the flour, cocoa powder, baking powder and salt. Set this aside.
2. Pour the THC oil and the chopped chocolate into a double boiler over high heat. As the water boils in the lower pan, whisk the chocolate and oil until melted. Remove from the heat, and whisk in the corn syrup, brown sugar and applesauce. Stir in the vanilla and egg whites. Beat the mixture until smooth, and then stir in the flour mixture until you get a smooth consistency.
3. Grease a 9-by-13-inch baking pan. Pour the batter into the pan. Bake for 20 minutes. The brownies are ready when the center of the top is almost firm to the touch. Remove from the oven and let it cool on a wire rack. Enjoy these chocolate treats!

Laws[10]

Legal Status in US
     Under the federal law, the use, sale and possession of cannabis in the United States However, there is a lot of diversity among the states. Some states have decriminalized non-medical cannabis use, making the drug completely legal. While others have only created exemptions for medical cannabis use and some have The truth is this is changing on every ballot.

     In four states, Washington, Colorado, Oregon and Alaska, recreational use of marijuana is legal for both medical and non-medical use. In 2014, voters in the District of Columbia voters overwhelmingly approved a ballot initiative legalizing recreational-purpose marijuana, but Congress has already attempted to gut funding for program. It's future is up in the air.

     Overall, 23 states and the District of Columbia have passed laws that allow medical use of marijuana to some extent, and 14 states have taken steps to decriminalize it to some point. The changes are making possession punishable by fine and confiscation please check a state-by-state breakdown at the end of the book for more information.

     Some states and local governments are asking law enforcement agencies to limit enforcement of drug laws with respect to cannabis. All of these changes have greatly reduced the number of "simple possession" offenders sent to jail, since federal enforcement agents rarely target individuals for relatively minor offenses, but they still focus on large organizations to some extent. This is all very controversial because under the Supremacy Clause of the United States

Constitution, federal law preempts conflicting state and local laws.

--------------------------------- ⚜ ---------------------------------

Using Tech to Find Weed

Weedmaps is an online legal marijuana community that allows users to review and talk about cannabis strains and local dispensaries. The website is similar to Yelp and contains a database with over 3,000 medical marijuana dispensaries and 25,000 strains of cannabis. The company was launched in July 2008 by Justin Hartfield and Keith Hoerling.

The site attracts about 2 million monthly visitors and has annual revenue of $18 million. Weedmaps is widely considered the industry leader and premier medical marijuana site on the web, catering to the entire industry from patients to businesses and continues to see substantial growth.

The site has expanded to also include recreational dispensaries in states where marijuana is legal. In addition they have launched a mobile app.

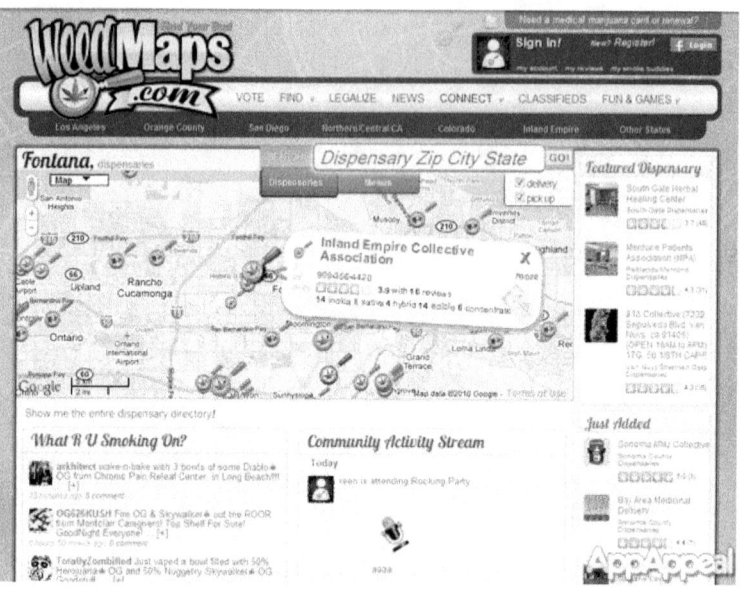

Reference Material

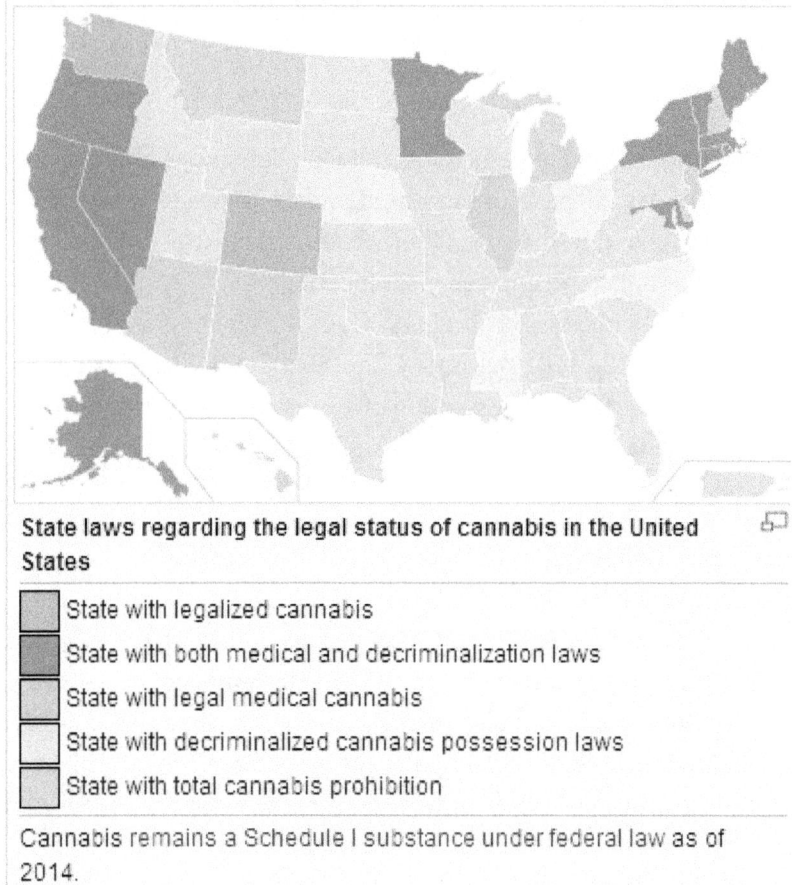

State laws regarding the legal status of cannabis in the United States

State with legalized cannabis

State with both medical and decriminalization laws

State with legal medical cannabis

State with decriminalized cannabis possession laws

State with total cannabis prohibition

Cannabis remains a Schedule I substance under federal law as of 2014.

Chart from: Website Title: Wikipedia Article Title: Cannabis in the United States

Alaska

In November, Alaska voters approved an initiative legalizing recreational marijuanafor those 21 years of age or older. The law will be enacted sometime in mid-Feburary of 2015, at which point it will be legal to be in possession of six plants, three of which can be mature, or possess or transport up to one ounce of weed.

California

California has one of the most detailed definitions of marijuana. It includes "all parts of the plant Cannabis sativa L., whether growing or not; the seeds thereof; the resin extracted from any part of the plant; and every compound, manufacture, salt, derivative, mixture, or preparation of the plant, its seeds, or its resin." (H&SC 11018). Under California Health & Safety Code as of January 1, 2011, possession of 1 ounce (28 g) or less of marijuana is an infraction, punishable by a maximum $100 fine plus additional fees with no impact on criminal record.

Possession of loftier amounts of marijuana is classified as a misdemeanor punishable by up to $500 and six months in jail under Health & Safety Code. Possession of hashish or concentrated cannabis is an optional misdemeanor or felony, referred to as a wobbler. First and second time possession-only offenders may choose a treatment program instead of jail. Upon successful completion of the program, their conviction is erased. Possession (and personal use cultivation) offenders can also avoid conviction by making a plea deal..

Any sort of sale, transportation or distribution of marijuana is a felony under Health and Safety Code Sections. However for amounts one ounce or less transporting or giving away is a misdemeanor punishable by a maximum $100 fine. Do not sell or distribute to minors as it is a felony .

Cultivation of any amount of marijuana is a felony under Health and Safety Code, unless you are growing for personal use, but there must be no evidence of intent to sell. Unlike other states, there are no limits to personal use cultivation, but you must not have anything that appears you are selling.

Like alcohol or other drugs, it is illegal to drive while under the influence of marijuana. "Under the influence has been interpreted to imply some degree of impairment, not specific drugs. As noted above a driver that is found with 1 ounce in their vehicle are liable for a maximum $100 misdemeanor fine. Taking 1 toke does not necessarily mean you would receive a DUI, pending your impairment. Minors under the age of 21 convicted marijuana related offences will face a 12-month drivers license suspension, regardless of whether the offense was driving-related. Unlike federal law, California law requires a conviction for forfeiture of property involved in a drug crime. If 10 pounds or more are found vehicles may be forfeited under Health and Safety Code 11470.

Possession of medical marijuana is legal for medical patients and their designated primary. They are also allowed to cultivate (but not distribute or sell) marijuana. Keep in mind that medical marijuana patients are not protected while on federal park land or forest land in California. You should note there are reports of campers and those driving through federal land who are searched, and can be charged with federal possession statutes, and had the marijuana they had obtained under a state medical recommendation confiscated.] A California medical recommendation is not a defense in federal court to these charges.

Colorado

In 1975, Colorado passed a law which made possession of one ounce or less of the cannabis plant a second degree petty offense only punishable by a fine of 100 dollar. In 2005, thirty years later, the city of Denver passed a new law which allowed adults over 21 to possess up to one ounce of marijuana without penalty in the city.

But the state of Colorado still imposed penalties for use and possession of marijuana.

In November 2012, Marijuana Policy Project backed the Campaign to Regulate Marijuana Like Alcohol, and successfully passed Amendment 64, making Colorado the first place in the world to have legalized possession, use, production, distribution, and personal cultivation of marijuana. The Marijuana Policy Project also played a chief role in drafting and campaigning for the important initiative.

Its worth noting that the amendment more support, than votes for President Obama. In downtown Denver there has been an explosion of legal pot shops. Many of these take cash only as national banks will not work with them for fear of losing their FDIC insurance. It will remain illegal to be found driving under the influence of marijuana, while legal possession will be limited to over-21s only and quantities regulated. Growing up to six plants will be legal, while it will also be legal to give away small quantities.

Connecticut

Governor Dan Malloy of Connecticut, On June 30, 2011, signed legislation into law decriminalizing the possession of small, personal use amounts of marijuana by adults. The law took effect on July 1 2011.

Senate Bill 1014 reduces the penalties for the adult possession of up to one-half ounce of marijuana from a criminal misdemeanor (formerly punishable by one year in jail and a $1,000 fine) are now a non-criminal infraction, punishable by a, no arrest or jail time, $150 fine, and no impact to criminal record. The new law similarly reduces penalties for the possession of marijuana paraphernalia.

Possession of larger amounts of marijuana is still illegal and punishable by imprisonment and monetary fines. A subsequent offense of possession of one-half ounce of marijuana is still a non- criminal infraction but the fine rises to $200–$500. First offense of possessing one-half to four ounces is a misdemeanor punishable by up to one year in prison and $1,000 in fine. Keep in mind that another offense becomes a felony punishable by with up to 5 years in jail and $3,000 fine.

First offense of possession of 4 ounces or more is a felony punishable by 5 years imprisonment and $2,000 fine. Subsequent offenses are punishable by 10 years in jail and a fine of $5,000. The minimum mandatory sentence for possession of marijuana within 1,500 feet of a school is 2 years' in jail, that will be added to other required jail time.

Selling any amount of marijuana is completely illegal and a felony punishable by no less than 7 years in jail and $25,000 in fine. Selling to minors and possessing within 1,500 feet of a school or day care are both felonies which adds 3 years imprisonment to any other sentence imposed. There's no monetary fine imposed.

On June 1, 2012, Governor Dan Malloy signed House Bill No. 5389, which allows the use of cannabis for certain "debilitating medical conditions."

District of Columbia

In November 2014, Voters in D.C. approved Initiative 71, which allows for the possession of up to two ounces of pot and home cultivation of up to three mature cannabis plants. But a pending deal reached by Congress in December could prohibit the District from legalizing marijuana for much of 2015. District officials have said that the deal reached by Congress does not carry the legal power to prevent them from implementing legalized marijuana.

Florida

A constitutional amendment sponsored by People United for Medical Marijuana obtained 745,613 signatures by Jan. 24, 2014 (683,149 were required by Feb. 1). The Supreme Court in Florida ruled 4-3 in favor of allowing the initiative to be decided by voters in the November election, which was decided on January 27, 2014.

B20 409 replaced the penalty for possession of up to one ounce of marijuana with a $25 civil fine. It was approved by the D.C. Council on March 4, signed by Mayor Vincent Gray on March 31, and became law on July 17 after surviving a Congressional review period. On November 4, voters approved Initiative 71, which will legalize possession and cultivation of limited amounts of marijuana for adults 21 and older. The measure will only go into effect after surviving a Congressional review period.

Illinois

The Illinois General Assembly passed the Compassionate Use of Medical Cannabis Pilot Program Act in 2013, which was signed by Governor Pat Quinn on August 1. The law legalizes the use of medical cannabis in tightly controlled circumstances. "Legally registered patients" may, with a prescription from a medical caregiver, apply for an ID card that allows the use of marijuana for medical purposes.

Maine

Possession of less than 2.5 oz (71 g) is a civil violation, punishable by a fine of $200–400. Possession of 2.5 oz (71 g) or more is considered evidence of intent to distribute and is punished as such. Possession of a usable amount of marijuana is lawful if at the time of the possession the person has an authenticated copy of a medical record demonstrating that the person has a physician's recommendation. Possession of greater than one pound of marijuana is considered trafficking and is punishable by up to one year in jail and a fine of up to $2,000.

Cultivation of five plants or less of marijuana is punishable by up to six months in jail and a fine of up to $1,000. For greater than five plants, the penalties increase to up to one year in jail and a fine of up to $2,000. For greater than 100 plants the possible punishment is up to five years in prison and a fine of up to $5,000. For any amount of plants greater than 500, the penalties increase to up to ten years in prison and a fine of up to $20,000.

The penalty for sale of marijuana is up to one year in jail and a fine up to $2,000. The penalties increase to up to five years in prison and a fine of up to $5,000 if the sale was made to a minor or if it occurred within 1,000 ft (300 m) of a school or on a school bus.

Possession and personal use of paraphernalia is a civil violation punishable by a fine of $200. The sale of paraphernalia is punishable by up to six months in prison and a fine of up to $1,000, unless the sale was to a minor, in which case the penalty increases to up to one year in jail and a fine of up to $2,000. Upon conviction, the court may suspend or revoke the professional license of the offender.

Maryland

Possession of less than 10 grams of marijuana in Maryland is punishable by a fine of up to $500 and 90 days in jail.

A proposed bill that would remove all criminal and civil penalties for the possession of up to one ounce of marijuana, allow the personal cultivation of up to 6 marijuana plants by those over the age of 21 and create a system of retail marijuana stores, cultivation facilities, and marijuana product manufacturers is due to be introduced into legislation in early 2014.

Massachusetts

In 2008, Massachusetts voters approved a ballot initiative to decriminalize a possession of up to an ounce of marijuana, and in 2009, ALM GL ch. 94C, § 32L was enacted into law, making possession of up to one ounce of marijuana a civil offense punishable by a penalty of $100 and forfeiting the drug. There are no other forms of civil or criminal punishments for offenders who are over 18 years of age.

In 2012, Massachusetts voters approved another ballot initiative to legalize possession and use of marijuana for medical purposes. The law puts medical marijuana under the jurisdiction of the state Department of Public Health, which is charged with setting up registration for patients and dispensaries and monitoring the business. Under the law, patients are allowed to possess a sixty-day supply (to be defined by the DPH) and appoint a representative to facilitate their use if they are incapable. The DPH is required to register at least one dispensary per county with a state-wide limit of 35.

Possession of more than one ounce of marijuana is a misdemeanor resulting into a $500 fine and up to six months' imprisonment with probation, after which records are sealed. Subsequent offenses are subjected to the same punishments but records are not sealed after probation.

The sale of less than 50 pounds of marijuana is a misdemeanor punishable by two years in prison with probation and a $5,000 fine. Subsequent offenders are subjected to up to 2½ years in prison without probation and a fine of $1,000–$10,000. Selling of more than 50 pounds is a felony punishable by 2½–15 years incarceration atop the minimum mandatory sentence (MMS).

 The MMS for selling up to 100 lbs is one year incarceration plus a fine of $500–$10,000. The MMS for selling 100–2000 lbs of marijuana is 3–15 years in prison and a fine of $2,500–$25,000. The MMS for selling 2000–10,000 lbs of marijuana is 5–15 years plus a fine of $5,000–$50,000 and that of selling more than 10,000 lbs of marijuana is 10–15 years incarceration plus up to $200,000 in fine. Selling marijuana within 1,000 feet of a school or 100 feet of a park is also a felony punishable by two years imprisonment in addition to the MMS and a fine of $1,000–$1,000.

Michigan

In the November election of 2008, more than 60% of Michigan voters supported Proposal 1, and Michigan thereby became the thirteenth state to legalize medical cannabis. On 4 December 2008, the Michigan Medical Marihuana Act was enacted, allowing patients with debilitating medical conditions such as HIV, cancer, and Hepatitis C to legally possess and use cannabis. The patient can have up to two and a half ounces of usable cannabis, and twelve plants kept in an enclosed and locked facility.

Recreational use of marijuana has not been decriminalized in the state of Michigan. However, most cities have decriminalization laws. Possession of any amounts of the plant is a misdemeanor punishable by up to one year incarceration and a $2,000 fine, while actual using is punishable by up to 90 days in jail and a $100 fine. If possession is in a public park, the sentence is at most 2 years and a $2,000 fine. Distributing marijuana without remuneration is a misdemeanor punishable by at most one year in jail and a $1,000 fine.

The sale and cultivation of cannabis is a felony punishable by up to 4–15 years imprisonment and $20,000-$10,000,000 in fines depending on the number of plants grown and the amount of usable cannabis sold.

Minnesota

On May 29,2014 Minnesota legalized medical marijuana, making it the twenty-second state to do so. It is considered to be the most restrictive medical marijuana bill in the country. Smoking actual plant material is illegal. Vapors, oils, and pills are the only legal forms of consumption.

Missouri

House Bill 2238, "Allows the Department of Agriculture to grow industrial hemp for research purposes and allows the use of hemp extract to treat certain individuals with epilepsy." The bill demands a neurologist to determine that the "intractable epilepsy" does not respond to at least three treatment options for a person to be eligible to use the marijuana extract. HB 2238 only allows hemp extract that contains more than 5% of cannabidiol (CBD) and no more than 0.3% tetrahydrocannabinol (THC).

New Hampshire

Currently, under New Hampshire state law, it is considered a misdemeanour to possess any amount of marijuana, subject to incarceration of up to 1 year and a maximum fine of $2000.

On the 15 January 2014 New Hampshire's legislature voted 170 to 162 in favor of 'House Bill 492', based on Colorado Amendment 64, which seeks to legalize under state law the personal use of up to one ounce of marijuana by persons 21 years of age or older and establish regulations for the retail production and sale of cannabis. The vote to approve the bill is the first time a chamber of a state legislature has ever approved of legislation to legalize and regulate marijuana for all adults. Tax issues pertaining to the bill are yet to be debated and a second House floor vote is expected in early 2014.

New York

In 1977, the state of New York also passed a law which decriminalized marijuana to a large extent. Possession of 25 g (0.88 oz) or less of marijuana, first offense, is a civil citation with a fine of $100 and the fine is increased to $200 for second offense. A third offense is a misdemeanor and the offender may get 5 days in jail and or pay $250 in fine. Possession of up to 2 ounces of marijuana is also a misdemeanor punishable by 3 months in jail and $500 in fines. Possession of 2 to 8 ounces (57 to 227 g) of marijuana is a class A misdemeanor that may be punishable by 1 year in jail or a $1000 fine or both. Possession of up to 16 oz (450 g) of marijuana is a class E felony punishable by 1–4 years in jail and a fine of $5000. Repeat offenders are mandated 6 months in jail plus a $5000 fine and/or an additional 3–4 years in jail. Possession of up to 10 lb (4.5 kg) of marijuana is a class D felony which is punishable by up to 15 years in jail and/or a fine of $5000 and second offenders must be incarcerated for at least 6 months. Possession of more than 10 lb (4.5 kg) is a class A felony also punishable by up to 15 years in jail and/or $5000 fine.

Selling or cultivation The selling of marijuana or cultivation of cannabis can be punished by prison sentences and fines which can vary with nature of the offence.

2 oz (57 g) or less is a class B misdemeanor punishable by jail time of 3 months and/or a fine of $500.

24 g (0.85 oz) sale is class A misdemeanor punishable by 1 year and/or $1,000 fine.

25 g (0.88 oz) to 4 oz (110 g) (first offense) is a class E felony punishable by 1–4 years and/or $5000 fine.

Second time offenders must do at least half jail sentence.

4 to 16 ounces (110 to 450 g) (first offense) is a class D felony punishable by 1–7 years in jail or $5000 fine (Possible probation if no prior felony offenses).

16 oz (450 g) to 10 lb (4.5 kg) (first offense) is a class C felony punishable by 1–5 years and/or fine of $5000.

Second offense time offenders must serve at least half the jail sentence.

10 lb (4.5 kg) or more (first offense) is a class C felony punishable by 1–15 years in jail and/or $5000 fine.

Second offense gives 6–15 years prison sentence and must serve at least half the jail sentence.

Sale to a minor is a class D felony punishable by 1–7 years in jail plus a $5,000 fine.

Oregon

In November 2014, Oregon voters overwhelming approved Measure 91, which will legalize the possession, private use, and cultivation of marijuana by adults 21 and older. The law will kick in on July 1, 2015. Oregon has a long history of tolerating marijuana. In 1973, Oregon became the first state to decriminalize cannabis. Possession of 28.35 grams (1 ounce) or less is a violation (not a crime) punishable by a $500 to $1,000 fine. Possession of 1 ounce to 110 grams is punishable by 10 years in prison, and possession of more than 110 grams is a felony with punishment depending on the defendant's prior record. In 1998, Oregon voters legalized medical marijuana through Oregon Ballot Measure 67 (1998).

Washington

In November 2012 Initiative 502 passed by Washington voters with 55.7% voting for the measure, and 44.3% against. This initiative will allow adults over the age of 21 to legally possess up to 1 ounce (28 g) of marijuana, 16 oz (450 g) of marijuana infused product in solid form, 72 oz (2.0 kg) of marijuana infused product in liquid form or any combination of all three and to legally consume marijuana, and marijuana infused products.

Wisconsin

The possession, sale and usage of marijuana in Wisconsin is currently illegal under state law. In April 2014 Wisconsin legalized CBD, a non-psychoactive marijuana extract oil, to treat children with severe epilepsy. On April 1, 2014 voters of Dane county voted on a nonbinding referendum to legalize marijuana. It passed with 65% of the vote.

Weed Dictionary[11]

Acapulco Gold: Marijuana strain from Acapulco, Mexico noted for its orange and gold hairs.

Aluminum pipe: A smoking utensil made from aluminum.

Apple pipe: A smoking utensil made from an apple.

Aqua lung: A gravity bong in a bucket.

Ash: 1. The solid waste left in a pipe after the combustion of useful marijuana. 2. The act of clearing waste from a smoking utensil.

Ashed: An empty bowl.

Auto: A smoking device consisting of an aquarium pump and an oxygen mask.

Babysitting: Holding smoke for too long.

Baggie: Any size plastic bag used for containing marijuana.

Bake break: To take a break from all activities and smoke marijuana.

Baked: To be heavily "inspired" by the consumption of cannabis.

Bake sale: A marijuana smoking session.

Bale: A compressed brick of marijuana.

Bing: Water pipe / bong.

Binger: Water pipe / bong.

Biz-ong: Water pipe / bong.

Black: Hash.

Blazed: Very high on marijuana.

Blitzed: Very high on marijuana.

Blow-back: To exhale smoke into someone's mouth. AKA – "shot gun".

Blunt: A cigar-sized joint usually rolled using cigar paper.

Bogart: Taking numerous hits before passing the smoking utensil without the consent of the circle or group.

Bong: A water pipe.

Bongmaster: Keeper and "packer" of the bong.

Bong rip: To take a hit from a bong.

Bong water: Water used in a water pipe to filter smoke.

Bootie: Another word for pirate treasure.

Bowl: 1. The end of a pipe in which weed is loaded. 2. A small amount of marijuana. 3. A packed bowl of marijuana.

Braindead: Loss of mental acuity.

Brainfart: Temporary loss of mental acuity.

Brick: A kilogram-sized slab or cube of compressed pot.

Bubblegum: 1. A term used to describe the smell or taste of marijuana. 2. When the weed is so sticky you have to cut it with scissors or a knife.

Bud: 1. The part of the cannabis plant you smoke. 2. The fresh or dried flowers of the female marijuana plant.

Buddha stick: A potent strain of grass from Thailand, usually wrapped around thin bamboo splints or Popsicle stick slivers.

Buds: A natural cluster of smokable marijuana.

Bucket bong: Any pipe using water and gravity to force the smoke into the "toker's" lungs. AKA – Gravity bong.

Bunk: Poor quality weed, usually containing numerous seeds.

Burn: 1. To act of smoking weed. 2. The sometimes exhausting after effects of smoking marijuana.

Burner: One who smokes marijuana then becomes complacent to do nothing.

Burnout: To suffer physical and mental exhaustion when coming down from a "high".

Burnt out: Complete physical and mental exhaustion.

Buzz: A mild cannabis high.

Buzz kill: A person or event that lessens the state of one's "high" in a negative manner.

Cannabis Indica: The scientific name for a species of marijuana plant.

Cannabis Sativa: The scientific name for a species of marijuana plant.

Can pipe: A smoking utensil made from a can.

Carb: A hole in a pipe or bong that allows the smoke to clear from the chamber and into your lungs.

Cashed: When the marijuana in the bowl of a smoking utensil has become primarily ash.

Chamber: 1. The longest section of a bong that holds smoke. 2. Pipe pieces formed to store and resonate weed.

Cherried: A continuous burning of the weed in a pipe, bong, or joint.

Cherry: The burning portion of weed that stays lit without further ignition.

Chillum: A cone-shaped pipe made of clay, the earliest form of smoking, originated from using a horn.

Chronic: An excellent quality marijuana.

Chronie: See "Chronic."

Circles: Circular groups formed by multiple pot smokers during a session.

Clogged: When it becomes difficult to suck through a smoking utensil.

Colombian: The most common type of grass on the black market.

Cool: 1. High. 2. Awesome. 3. Thanks.

Cornering: Lighting only a portion of the bowl at a time so that more than one person can get a green hit.

Cottonmouth: A lack of saliva brought about by smoking marijuana.

Crash: To lose your energy fast and hard after smoking marijuana.

Creeper: Weed that takes time to alter your state of mind after being inhaled.

Dank: High-quality marijuana.

Deal: An illegal cannabis purchase.

De-childproof: To remove the child-safety devise.

De-seeding: Removing all stems and seeds from a quantity of marijuana.

Dime: A quantity of weed costing ten dollars.

Dirt: Poor quality weed, usually containing numerous seeds.

Doobie: A joint.

Dope: 1. Marijuana. 2. Name given to any illegal substance. 3. Cool, awesome.

Dry: When you and/or your hook-up run out of marijuana.

Dub: A quantity of weed costing twenty dollars.

Eighth: One-eighth ounce of marijuana.

Elbow joint: A pipe piece that connects the chamber and bowl.

Euro-style: Taking multiple hits before passing the smoking utensil with the consent of the circle or group.

Faded: 1. A term used to describe a state of being high. 2. Feeling too high.

Fatty: A very thick joint.

Fish-lipping: Using excessive saliva while smoking from a joint or pipe.

Five-O: Police (as in Hawaii Five-O).

Four-twenty: The international time to smoke pot.

Fuzz: Police.

Ganja: Indian and Jamaican term for marijuana.

Grass: Marijuana, weed, pot, etc.

Gravity bong: Any pipe using water and gravity to force the smoke into the "toker's" lungs.

Green: 1. An excellent quality marijuana. 2. The basic color of marijuana.

Green hit: The first hit: refers to the color of marijuana.

Half "O": A half ounce of marijuana.

Harsh: Herb that is too dry and burns too fast.

Hash / Hashish: Hash is formed by scraping the sticky resin from the leaves of the marijuana plant.

Head change: The mental change that occurs from smoking marijuana, usually accompanied by an altered awareness of time.

Head shops: Any shop that sells marijuana-smoking paraphernalia.

Hemp: Cannabis stalks and stems, especially those used to make rope, fabrics, etc.

Hemp Wick: A thin hemp cord (fueled by beeswax) used for igniting marijuana.

Herb: Jamaican term for marijuana with Biblical connotations; Rastafarian sacrament.

High: The mental change that occurs from smoking marijuana, usually accompanied by an altered awareness of time.

Hit: The act of inhaling pot smoke into your lungs.

Hookah: A hashish waterpipe with four long stems to accommodate four smokers at once, originates back to the Middle East.

Hook-up: The person from whom you get your weed.

House rules: Rules set by the host to be followed during all gatherings and parties.

Hot box: To smoke weed inside a vehicle with the widows rolled up.

Hydro: Hydroponically grown marijuana.

"I'm Cool": 1. "I have had enough to smoke." 2. "I do not wish to smoke." 3."I'm high."

Indica: Type of marijuana.

Indo: Marijuana, term from Northern California

J / Jay: A joint.

Joint: A marijuana cigarette.

Jonesing: A need for drugs.

Kaff / Khayf / Kif / Kief: Golden pollen hash from Morocco, Lebanon and other Arab/Middle Eastern nations. Common forms are Red Lab and Slate.

Kind: High quality marijuana.

Lagger: A person who seemingly takes forever to do everything.

Light: A lighter or match.

Light up: The act of lighting marijuana.

Lip burner: A pipe that is too short for practical use.

Lit: The state of being high.

Load a bowl: Loading a pipe or bong with marijuana.

Lung-cookie: A coughed up ball of phlegm.

Marijuana: The smokable leaves and buds of the female cannabis plant.

Mary Jane: The female cannabis plant. Male plants have almost no active THC.

Mex: A description of poor quality weed often imported from Mexico.

Mexy: See "Mex."

Mooching: Always smoking other people's weed, but never supplying it.

Mouthpiece: The end of the pipe which is placed between your lips as you smoke.

Mush brain: Extreme mental fatigue associated with "coming down" from your high.

Munch: To eat without thinking.

Munchies: The hunger sensation associated with being high.

Nickel: 1. 0.5 grams of marijuana 2. 1/2 gram.

Nipple: The mouthpiece of a pipe.

NORML: An organization for the rights of pot smokers.

Northern Lights: An extremely high-grade marijuana.

Nug: A bud from a marijuana plant or a part there of.

"O": One ounce of marijuana.

Oil: The purified and concentrated resin from hashish or marijuana.

O-ring: Small rubber rings that help create an airtight seal between pipe pieces.

O.Z.: One ounce of marijuana.

Ounce: One ounce of marijuana.

Pack a bowl: Load a smoking utensil with marijuana.

Party foul: A breaking of basic house rules, such as knocking over a bong or loading a seed.

Peanut: What is left of a joint after it has become so small that it's difficult to smoke. It is strong because it catches and concentrates the resin of the joint.

Piece: Used to describe any smoking utensil.

Pinner: A very thin joint.

Pipe: A tubular implement used for smoking marijuana.

Poker: Any device used to clear a smoking utensil of ash and resin.

Pot: Marijuana, hash, grass, cannabis, etc.

Pot brownies: Brownies laced with marijuana or THC.

Pot-butter / Cannabutter: Butter infused with marijuana.

Pound: One pound of marijuana.

Pretendo: 1. Marijuana that looks and smells excellent, but does not deliver a great high. 2. Prematurely picked marijuana.

Puff-puff-give: Taking only one or two tokes before passing the hit.

Puff-puff-pass: See "Puff-puff-give."

Q.P.: A quarter pound (four ounces) of marijuana.

Quarter: 1. A quarter ounce of marijuana. 2. A quarter pound of marijuana.

Reefer: And old-school term meaning marijuana.

Resin: A sticky brown residue deposited in smoking utensils via combustion of marijuana.

Resonate: To strengthen and concentrate your weed.

Roach: What is left of a joint after it has become so small that it's difficult to smoke. It is strong because it catches and concentrates the resin of the joint.

Roach-clip: A device for holding a roach.

Roller: A device used to facilitate joint rolling.

Rolling paper: Thin paper used to form marijuana cigarettes.

Sack: Any measurement of weed contained within baggie.

Salad Bowl: When you pack a bowl beyond the lip of the bowl itself.

Scale: Any of various measuring tools used to weigh out marijuana.

Score: 1. A 70's term for a quarter ounce of hash. 2. To receive and / or purchase marijuana.

Screen: A metal or glass filter designed to let smoke through and keep ash out.

Seed: The seed from a fertilized marijuana plant.

Session: Two or more pot-smokers gathered for a common purpose: to get high.

Shake: The very small and dry pieces of marijuana used in the joint rolling process.

Sinsemilla: The flowering tops of seedless plants.

Sinker: A bowl that usually does not require a screen.

Skunk: 1. Aromatic and potent sinsemilla.2. A term used to describe the quality or fragrance of marijuana.

Smoke: 1. To light and inhale marijuana smoke. 2. Pot, reefer, grass, etc.

Smoke break: To stop what you are doing a smoke weed.

Smoking circle: A gathering of persons smoking pot.

Smoking utensil: Any device used to smoke marijuana.

Snap: To completely empty the bowl of a water pipe by sucking though it.

Spark it: Light up.

Spliff: A Jamaican term for a large cone-shaped joint.

Stash: A personal supply of marijuana.

Stem: 1. The cylinder on a bong that connects the chamber to the bowl. 2. The stem from a marijuana plant.

Stoned: The state of being high.

Stoney: 1. Cool. 2. A nice quality weed.

Stress: Poor quality weed, usually containing numerous seeds.

Stuck: Being unaware and unable to process complex thoughts.

THC / Tetrahydrocannabinol: The psychoactive cannabinoid element in cannabis that is responsible for the "high".

Thai stick: A potent strain of grass from Thailand, usually wrapped around thin bamboo splints or Popsicle stick slivers.

Toke: Taking a hit from a smoking utensil.

Toker: One who smokes marijuana.

To your head: 1. "Finish the bowl yourself." 2. "You took a really big hit."

Triple beam: A type of scale with great accuracy.

Utensil: A device such as a bong or pipe used to smoke marijuana.

Vaporizer: A device that heats your marijuana to the exact "vaporizing" temperature of the active chemicals.

Visine: A brand name eye drop.

Visual: An hallucination.

Wake and bake: To smoke weed upon waking up.

Wasted: Stoned beyond rational thought.

Water pipe: A device used to filter marijuana smoke through water before it is inhaled.

Weed: Marijuana.

White Widow: A name given to many varieties of great marijuana with a white crystalline appearance.

X: Ecstasy

Yellow Taxi: A yellow-haired weed typically grown in Amsterdam.

Z: 1 ounce of cannabis.

Zigzag: A name brand rolling paper

Zoned: A loss of the ability to focus on more than one thing at a time.

Special thanks to all that support and encourage me to follow my crazy ideas. Thanks to my editor David, pleasure working with you. Frank, let me know if you ever have the munchies. Kurt thanks for going on the adventure to Colorado with me. Geoff and Zak you were on the couch last night, it was cool. Paige you are sitting by me and have no idea what I am working on.

Bibliography

1. Website Title: Buzzle

Article Title: Different Types of Weed and Their Effects

Publisher: Buzzle.com

Date Accessed: September 16, 2014

Author: Rahul Thadani

http://www.buzzle.com/articles/different-types-of-weed-and-their-effects.html

2. Website Title: Marijuana

Article Title: Guide to Smoking Weed

Date Accessed: September 16, 2014

http://marijuana.com/community/threads/guide-to-smoking-weed.190395/

3. Website Title: WebMD

Article Title: Recreational Marijuana: Are There Health Effects?

Publisher: WebMD

Date Accessed: September 16, 2014

Author: Kathleen Doheny

http://www.webmd.com/smoking-cessation/news/20121207/recreational-marijuana-health-effects

4. Website Title: FC Vaporizer Review Forum
Article Title: Sublimation
Date Accessed: September 16, 2014
http://fuckcombustion.com/threads/sublimation.9783/

5. Website Title: Wikipedia
Article Title: Cannabis foods
Publisher: Wikimedia Foundation
Electronically Published: August 09, 2014
Date Accessed: September 16, 2014
http://en.wikipedia.org/wiki/Cannabis_foods

6. Website Title: How to Cook with Weed
Article Title: Cooking with weed
Date Accessed: September 16, 2014
http://www.thestonerscookbook.com/how_to_cook_with_wee
d.php

7. Website Title: The Stoner's Cookbook
Article Title: Special Brownies
Date Accessed: September 16, 2014
http://www.thestonerscookbook.com/recipe/special-brownies

8. Website Title: The Price of Weed, Marijuana, Cannabis
Article Title: What is Marijuana really worth?
Date Accessed: September 16, 2014
http://www.priceofweed.com/

9. Website Title: Grow Cannabis

Article Title: Introduction To Growing Cannabis

Date Accessed: September 16, 2014

http://growcannabis.weebly.com/

10. Website Title: Wikipedia

Article Title: Cannabis in the United States

Publisher: Wikimedia Foundation

Electronically Published: September 14, 2014

Date Accessed: September 16, 2014

http://en.wikipedia.org/wiki/Cannabis_in_the_United_States

11. Website Title: Smoking With Style Pot Dictionary
Comments

Article Title: Pot Dictionary, Marijuana Terms

Date Accessed: September 16, 2014

http://www.smokingwithstyle.com/pot-etiquette/pot-dictionary/

www.ingramcontent.com/pod-product-compliance
Lightning Source LLC
Chambersburg PA
CBHW071002180526
45168CB00003B/1260